Kundalini Yoga:

A Meditation Awakening Guide for Beginners

By: Alyson Rodgers

Published by:
Alyson Rodgers and Random Technologies
4409 HOFFNER AVENUE, 347
Orlando, FL 32812

www.SparrowPublications.com

Table of Contents

Introduction

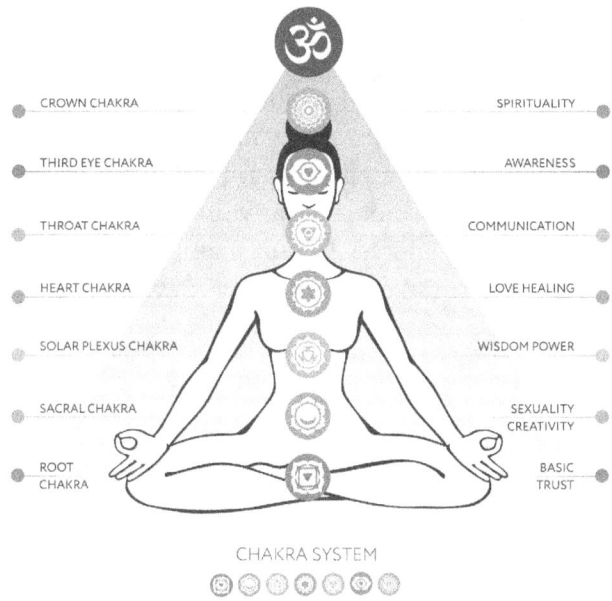

CROWN CHAKRA SPIRITUALITY

THIRD EYE CHAKRA AWARENESS

THROAT CHAKRA COMMUNICATION

HEART CHAKRA LOVE HEALING

SOLAR PLEXUS CHAKRA WISDOM POWER

SACRAL CHAKRA SEXUALITY CREATIVITY

ROOT CHAKRA BASIC TRUST

CHAKRA SYSTEM

Are you looking for increased happiness, well-being, and mental clarity? Do you want to let go of negative thought? This is and more is possible with kundalini yoga.

Through a combination of breathing techniques, hand gestures, mantras, meditation, and asanas, you can awaken the energy that lies dormant within your body.

This energy moves through your body and consciousness. Yet, many people never harness it. You can improve your health through this ancient practice and feel a surge of energy, unlike anything you have experienced before.

Kundalini yoga is considered **the mother of all yoga**, as it incorporates various techniques, such as body poses, breathing techniques, meditation, and chanting. It is the complete yoga for the mind and body and offers numerous benefits.

How do you get started? By reading this introduction to kundalini yoga. Discover answers to the most important questions:

- What is kundalini yoga?
- What are the benefits of this practice?
- How do you begin practicing kundalini yoga?

Kundalini yoga is **great for men and women of all ages**. Use this guide, as your introduction to kundalini yoga. Find out how to awaken the wasted energy within your body. Clear your mind, promote creativity, remove negativity, and increase your happiness through kundalini yoga. Get started today and begin working towards a better tomorrow.

What is Kundalini?

There are many different types of yoga and kundalini yoga is one of these branches. Though, unlike other forms of yoga, kundalini yoga focuses on more than just the body. It is the complete yoga – paying equal attention to the well-being of your body and your mind.

What exactly is kundalini? The name itself comes from "kundal", a Sanskrit word for spiral or coil. In this sense, kundalini can be thought of as coiled power – as in a serpent that lies coiled. The power is resting – waiting to be awakened.

Kundalini is an energy, while **kundalini yoga is the practice** of awakening this energy. Through various poses, breathing, chanting, and meditation, kundalini yoga can help you improve physically, spiritually, and mentally.

How Is Kundalini Yoga Different from Other Forms of Yoga?

When people think of yoga, they often picture the various poses. These poses are referred to as asanas. They are an important part of kundalini yoga, but there are additional practices involved in kundalini yoga.

With kundalini yoga, you will perform a kriya. A kriya is basically a series of techniques put together to help change your mind, body, and spirit at the same time. You will awaken energy in order to help with physical and mental changes.

These techniques include the following:

- Asanas (postures)
- Pranayama (special breathing, including Breath of Fire)
- Mudras (hand gestures)

- Bhandas (body locks)
- Mantras (chanting)
- Meditation

This guide will give instruction in all of these areas. You will learn which kriya to use for specific purposes. This includes kriya for dealing with headaches, kriya for mental clarity and focus, or simply for improved health and happiness.

Three Forms of Kundalini Energy

Prana is often described as the vital breath. It is the main universal energy and is commonly mentioned in yoga texts. This is the energy within you and around you.

With kundalini yoga, this is generally referred to as prana-kundalini. Prana-kundalini is just one of three forms of kundalini:

- Para-kundalini (un-manifested energy)
- Prana-kundalini (universal energy)
- Shakti-kundalini (manifested energy)

The para-kundalini is the universal energy, while the prana-kundalini is the mind/body energy. Shakti is the entire consciousness and bridges the gap between these other two manifestations.

Understanding Chakras and the Granthis

Your body contains a series of chakras. These **chakras are points of energy** located throughout your body. When chakras are blocked by knots or other obstacles, the flow of energy, or prana, is blocked.

Kundalini yoga can help remove these knots, which are also referred to as Granthi. These blockages can prevent you from reaching your full potential. These knots can restrict instincts, block energy, and limit your awareness.

In kundalini yoga, there are three common Granthis in your central pathway that can prevent you from awakening kundalini:

- Brahma Granthi
- Vishnu Granthi
- Rudra Granthi

Brahma Granthi

Also known as the perineal knot, the Brahma Granthi is located over the muladahara and svadhisthana chakras. It can block the energies that are linked with awareness, sexual desire, and instincts. Kundalini yoga can help open these knots and allow the muladahara and svadhisthana energies to flow freely – providing a sense of happiness.

You are also diverting sexual energy that remains stagnant within your body to your brain. This distilled sexual energy commonly interferes with judgment, reasoning, and thought. By allowing this energy to rise, you can truly open your mind and increase your spiritual and mental development.

Vishnu Granthi

Opening the Vishnu granthi is believed to help connect the internal energy with the external energy. By opening the energy blocked by the Vishnu granthi, you can remove anger, jealousy, and hatred. Instead of relying solely on the energy locked within, you are opening yourself to receive energy from the universe.

Rudra Granthi

When Rudra granthi blocks energy, it can promote a sense of ego. You tend to focus inwards. Removing this blockage can help improve mental and physical awareness. Unleashing the Ajna and Sahasrara chakras that are blocked by the Rudra granthi is also required to evolve the sixth sense – the third eye.

Opening the Flow of Prana

In order to remove these blockages, you will perform a series of kriya each day. In the following chapters, you will learn more about this kriya, including the various poses, chants, and breathing techniques that go along with them.

The Origins of Kundalini Yoga

Where does kundalini yoga come from? There have been references to kundalini dating back for hundreds of years.

As mentioned, the word "Kundal" means coiled. This refers to the coiled serpent, as well as the coils at the base of the spine. These coils are formed by a triangular bone called the Sacrum – which has also been thought sacred, holy, and powerful by a large variety of civilizations over the years.

References to kundalini are found throughout the ancient text. One of the earliest direct references appears in the self-titled, "Gyaneshwari", circa 1275AD. He wrote, "Kundalini is one of the greatest energies."

Gyaneshwari went on to write that when the kundalini begins to rise, "…unwanted impurities in the body disappear." This explains the process of awakening the kundalini and removing the blocked Granthi in order to improve physical health.

You can also find direct comparisons to similar concepts in other cultures and religions. This speaks to the universal concepts that are an integral part of kundalini.

Similar concepts and ideas have also occurred in various religions. The coiled energy that you are attempting to unleash has been called different names in different cultures.

For example, the Chinese refer to a chi or qi energy. This includes the same core principles as kundalini.

In the Holy Koran, the Prophet Mohammed Sahib speaks of the day of resurrection, stating that the "hands will speak". People sometimes feel a flow of energy through the hands as kundalini rises. Similarities can also be found in Christianity. In Luke 17:21, "The Kingdom of God is within you."

While different cultures have had similar concepts about an energy within you, kundalini directly addresses the benefits of unleashing this energy. It provides a way to actually open up the flow of energy (prana-kundalini) and open your mind to your surroundings.

As the popularity of yoga spread to the Western world, various groups, gurus, and teachers began promoting kundalini yoga. Swami Nigamananda introduced kundalini yoga to the greater world with the release of a book in 1935. In the 1960's and 1980's yoga saw another boost in widespread practice.

You can now find a wealth of information on kundalini yoga. It is no longer a fringe practice. If you are ready to reach a state of bliss and inner peace, then continue reading to learn how to get started with kundalini yoga.

The Benefits of Awakening Kundalini

Why should you consider practicing kundalini yoga? What are the main advantages of performing the various poses and breathing techniques associated with kundalini? Millions of people have found profound changes through kundalini.

As the kundalini energy ascends, you should experience a natural awakening of energy. This removes clouded judgment. It can **improve mental clarity**. You should find a renewed sense of self-awareness.

Some of the areas that have been addressed through kundalini include:

- Depression
- Lack of focus
- Anger
- Fatigue
- Anxiety
- And many other mental and physical impairments

As you become more aware of the energy within and around you, you will notice these symptoms gradually decrease. That is one of the main goals of kundalini yoga. Though, you need to realize that not everyone will get the same results. In Western medicine, this would be thought of as a holistic approach.

Yoga and other Eastern practices are often met with skepticism in the West. Yet, these practices remain popular all over the world. Millions of people from all walks of life practice kundalini yoga.

It is hard to deny that yoga of all forms can have a calming effect. This is known to have a positive effect on your physical and mental health.

You can naturally improve your blood circulation, allowing for a better flow of blood and oxygen to your body and brain. This addresses the root cause of many of the ailments listed above. Through kundalini, you can gain a better connection to your consciousness and expand your self-awareness. You can live a harmonious and happy life.

How long will it take to see results? This depends on your current state of mind, your willingness to accept the fundamentals of kundalini, and how much of yourself you devote to this practice. With regular practice, you may experience any of the following physical benefits:

- Boost your energy levels
- Increase your lung capacity
- Promote better blood circulation
- Lower your blood pressure

Though, these are debatable. The reason for that kundalini provides the potential for these benefits comes from the breathing techniques and generally improved well-being. Along with physical benefits, the calming effect of kundalini can also lead to mental benefits:

- Improve your happiness and creativity
- Eliminate negative thoughts and habits
- Gain control over your emotions

You can perform the kriya presented later in this guide every day, several times per day, or more often – depending on how much time you have available. Many people have commented that kundalini yoga helps them clear their mind. They feel refreshed and energized after performing a kriya.

Getting Started with Kundalini

Kundalini involves the use of kriya. These kriyas include a selection of practices that are intended to open the flow of energy and improve your health in various ways.

Each kriya will consist of a series of poses, mantras, and other practices. This may include:

- Asanas
- Pranayama
- Mudras
- Bandhas
- Mantras
- Meditation

Asanas

Asanas are postures or poses that are performed to help loosen your body and open up your chakras in order to promote the flow of prana. Typically, when performing a kriya, you will combine an asana with mudras, bandhas, pranayama, and mantras to help affect your entire body.

This is one of the main ways that kundalini varies from other forms of yoga. Instead of simply performing a series of asanas while focusing on your breathing, you may perform one or two asanas, with a greater focus on the variety of techniques described below.

You may be familiar with some of the most common asanas, such as downward dog and forward bends. Though, in kundalini yoga, these names are not often used. Instead, descriptive names, such as spinal twist or nerve stretch are used.

Asanas serve multiple purposes. As a form of exercise, asanas are used to isolate specific muscles and help **increase blood circulation**. Focusing on specific areas may also be used to help improve organ function or redirect energy.

In meditation, asanas are used to help created a connection between your mind and body. It makes it easier to block stimuli when you are positioned in certain ways. It also opens up the energy pathways or chakras.

Pranayama

Pranayama refers to special **breathing techniques**, such as the Breath of Fire. Your breath includes prana, which is the main life force or energy. While you cannot live without oxygen, you also cannot live without prana.

It is known that slowing your rate of breathing can help calm your mind and give you more control over your emotions. When you are angry, you are told to take a deep breath. This is thought to deliver oxygen to your brain, giving the opportunity to relax, reflect, and then react. The oxygen does play a part, but so does the flow of prana.

By learning how to make the connection between breathing and your mind, you need to actively focus on your breathing. This is the goal of pranayama. Your mind follows your breath and your body will follow your mind.

Breath of fire is one of the more common examples of pranayama. This technique requires practice and you may want to watch a video online of a trained practitioner to understand the full technique.

Essentially, you will pump your navel point (center of your belly) in and out while breathing through your nose. You will attempt to breathe rapidly through your nose and with practice you will be able to match this to the pumping in and out of your navel point.

Breath of Fire can help **improve your lung capacity,** while also removing mucus and debris from the lining of your lungs. Some believe this can help remove disease from the lungs and help detoxify your respiratory system.

You can perform Breath of Fire and other breathing techniques while performing your asanas, mantras, and meditation. Remember, it is the combination of these techniques that helps create the full effect and increase your chances of awakening kundalini.

Mudras

Mudras are hand gestures. There are many important points along your hands and fingers. These points are directly connected to your emotions and your kundalini.

Positioning your hand in certain ways can help give a clear message to your mind and body. Again, you are adding a technique in order to further make a connection between your mind and body. Here are a few examples of commonly used mudras:

- Gyan Mudra
- Shuni Mudra
- Surya Mudra
- Buddhi Mudra
- Pranam Mudra

Gyan Mudra – For Wisdom and Calmness

The most commonly recognized mudra is the Gyan Mudra (Seal of Knowledge). With this mudra, you will touch the tip of your index finger to the tip of your thumb. Your other three fingers will remain straight. This is supposed to help stimulate your mind – helping you become more receptive to wisdom and knowledge.

Shuni Mudra – For Patience and Reflection

The Shuni Mudra (Seal of Patience) can help you remain patient. It is intended to help you take responsibility for your life and actions. Touch the tip of your middle finger to the tip of your thumb, keeping the other three fingers straight.

Surya Mudra – For Energy and Health

Surya Mudra (Seal of Sun) encourages improved energy, health, and nerve strength. Touch the tip of your ring finger to the tip of your thumb. Keep your other three fingers straight.

Buddhi Mudra – For Mental Clarity

The Buddhi Mudra (Seal of Mental Clarity) can clear your mind, stimulate spiritual development, and help you communicate clearly. Touch the tip of your little finger with the tip of your thumb, while keeping the other three fingers straight.

Pranam Mudra

Pranam Mudra, or the Prayer Pose, is a little different than the other mudras. You will place both of your palms together, with your fingers touching, as if in prayer. Bring your thumbs up to your sternum. This is believed to help relieve pressure and help you reach a meditative state.

Bandhas

Bandhas are body locks. There are four main body locks, each of which can help direct prana in order to help heal your mind, body, and soul. The four Bandhas include:

- Neck lock
- Root lock
- Diaphragm lock
- Great lock

Neck Lock

The neck lock is one of the most basic locks. It can help stabilize your upper body, making it easier to focus on your breathing, mantras, and meditation. It also helps regulate blood pressure and minimize distractions during your kriya.

To perform the neck lock, you will lift your chest and sternum upward while lengthening the back of your neck. Lift your chin toward the back of your neck. As you perform this lock, you should try to keep your face, throat, and neck muscles relaxed.

Root Lock

The root lock is supposed to help stimulate the flow of energy and spinal fluid. It is a powerful body lock and should not be performed by women that are menstruating.

Contract and hold the muscles located around your anus. At the same time, contract and hold the muscles around your pelvic region – as if impeding the flow of urine. The last step is to contract the muscles of your lower abdomen. The combination of this three movement may require practice, especially the combination of the first two.

Diaphragm Lock

The diaphragm lock should be performed on an empty stomach. It can help massage your intestines and heart. It cleanses your body and is believed to promote patience and compassion.

In order to perform the diaphragm lock, you should inhale and then exhale completely. Lift your abdominal region upward and back towards your spine. Do not contract your navel point. Lift your chest while slowly lowering the spine forward.

When you are in the correct position, the front of your throat should be prominent. Hold this pose for 10 to 60 seconds without straining your muscles or body. Then, relax your muscles and slowly inhale without releasing the pose. Again, this body lock may require practice.

Great Lock

The great lock is a combination of the previous locks. So, you will only be able to perform it when you have mastered the other three bandhas. In order to perform the great lock, perform all of the other three locks at the same time.

The great lock can provide a wide range of physical benefits. This includes a rejuvenation of your glands and nerves, which is believed to aid in the process of unblocking knots. Others notice increased energy and vitality. It is also thought to help cure various ailments, such as menstrual cramps, intestinal issues, high blood pressure, and stomach problems.

Mantras

Mantras are phrases that you repeat – either out loud or in your mind. When spoken out loud, these mantras are performed as a type of chant. The goal of using a mantra is to become more in-tune with the surrounding energies. There is a frequency that is universal to all life.

Along with helping you become more connected with the universal energy, you are also targeting pressure points along the roof of your mouth. This can help promote a chemical reaction in your brain that allows you to reach a higher state of consciousness. This is part of the reason that mantras are key to awakening kundalini. Here are a couple of mantras that are frequently used in Kundalini yoga:

Sat Nam (Truth is my identity)

The purpose of this mantra is to promote the concept that the divine energy or consciousness is within everyone. You have kundalini within you.

OngNamo Guru DevNamo (I bow to the creative wisdom. I bow to the divine teacher within)

This next mantra helps you link your inner consciousness with the divine energy. It prepares you for the kriya and helps open your mind to positivity.

Meditation

Meditation is also a crucial aspect of kundalini. While performing breathing techniques, asanas, mantras, and mudras, you will focus your energies on meditation. The techniques listed above are all used to help you reach a better state of meditation.

One of the primary purposes of meditation is to cleanse your mind. When you are without distraction, your mind tends to wander. You may have pleasant thoughts, as well as angry or perverse thoughts.

Dwelling on these thoughts can poison your psyche and make it difficult to improve your spiritual development. Meditation is a way of letting these thoughts simply pass by without any thought or notice. When you practice meditation, you will gain more control over your thoughts. You will be able to allow thoughts and negativity to pass through your mind without disrupting your inner peace or sense of calm.

Meditation really does require practice. You can try this for yourself right now. Simply close your eyes and try to think of nothing. Almost immediately, random thoughts will begin entering your mind. You may think about what you ate earlier, what you are going to do later, the sound that you hear outside, or any other random thought. This makes it difficult to focus on the flow of energy within you.

When you first start practicing kundalini yoga, you should choose a quiet location. Choose a spot that is completely free of distraction. You should try to use the same location each day. This will help you reach a state of peace during your meditation.

With practice, you will be able to meditate anywhere. You will be able to use your training in your everyday life. You will be able to not let things get to you. Negative experiences will simply become experiences.

Everyday Kundalini Kriyas

Kundalini is an easy concept to understand. You have an energy within you and around you. The goal of kundalini is to help you become more aware and improve the flow of energy through your body.

In the previous chapter, you learned about the various methods that are used to practice kundalini, such as Bandhas and mudras. You will now put these methods into practice with a series of kriya.

How to Follow a Kriya

The kriya can be thought of as an exercise or series of actions. Each kriya includes a selection of the methods already discussed, including an asana and a mantra. Other practices may be included. This will depend on the kriya and the goal of the kriya.

You will discover a variety of kriya that you can use to promote better health and well-being. Each of these exercises can take anywhere from a few minutes to 20 minutes. Read through each of the kriyas and choose one or two that you would like to focus on. Once you get used to one or two kriyas, you can attempt other kriya or search for additional examples online.

You can use any of the kriya provided or choose which actions to perform based on the ailment or problem that is troubling you, such as:

- Depression
- Pain
- Disease
- Detoxification
- Energy

- Headaches
- Vitality
- Overall health and well-being

Depression

The first kriya that you will learn will help combat depression and increase your happiness. This exercise is referred to as the Reverse Adi Shakti Kriya. It can help remove anger, depression, and a sense of hopelessness.

First, sit in Easy Pose. This is a basic asana with your legs crossed, while seated on the floor. Keep your spine straight. Hold your right palm about six inches above your head. The palm is facing down, giving you a blessing. For your left arm, bend your elbow and hold your left arm up. Your left palm should face outward, with your thumb several inches in front of your left shoulder. With your left hand, you are blessing the world.

Keep your eyes closed and breath in long, slow, deep breaths. Inhale for 20 seconds and then hold for 20 seconds before exhaling for 20 seconds.

Maintain your breathing and hold the pose for 11 minutes. Inhale slowly and then move into the next position.

Remain seated as you extend your palms in front of you. Keep your arms parallel to the ground. Keep your eyes closed and resume your slow, deep breathing. Remain in this position for 3 minutes and then stretch your arms straight up towards the ceiling. Point your fingertips upwards.

Hold this for 3 minutes, while breathing slowly and deeply. Afterward, you can stretch your arms and slowly tighten all of your muscles. Hold for 10 seconds and then relax. That is all that is required for this first kriya.

The first time that you perform any of these kriyas, you can follow along while reading this guide. After several attempts, you should be able to remember the steps. This allows you to focus on meditating. If you have trouble concentrating, you can use either of the mantras provided in the previous chapter to help you meditate.

Pain

This next kriya is intended to help you deal with pain. You can help heal your central nervous system. You can train your mind and body to fight pain.

Sit in Easy Pose, with your spine straight. Use the neck lock. Stretch your arms out to both sides. Your left palm should face downward, while your right palm should face upward.

Position your fingers so that your middle and index finger are together and your ring and little finger are together. This is similar to the hand signal made famous by the Star Trek character Spock.

Inhale deeply through your mouth and exhale through your nose. You should try to slow your breathing so that you are only inhaling and exhaling three times per minute. This is 20 seconds per breath.

Hold this pose for 11 minutes. If are unable to hold this for 11 minutes, do not worry. With practice, it will become easier to maintain the asanas described in these pages.

When you are ready to finish the pose, you should inhale deeply through your mouth. Hold your breath and then stretch your arms as you stretch your spine upward. Exhale through your nose, repeat the stretch and then resume regular breathing.

Disease

You can also help prevent disease by performing specific kriyas. This next one is designed to increase your disease resistance. This can also help with digestion issues and relieve illnesses that are centered in the stomach.

Sit on your heels. Next, stretch your arms straight up towards the ceiling. Press your palms together. Inhale, and as you inhale, begin pumping your stomach. Continue pumping your navel point until you need to breathe. You can then relax and exhale.

Repeat this process, of inhaling and pumping your stomach, for several minutes. This stimulates digestion.

Next, sit on your heels and place your hands in a bear grip in front of your chest. The bear grip is two hands interlocked. One palm should face your chest while the other faces outward. Inhale and hold your breath. Attempt to pull your hands apart. Exhale and then inhale before trying to pull your hands apart again. Repeat this process for several minutes.

You will now move your hands behind your back. Instead of interlocking them in a grip, you place them in a together with both palms facing your neck. Inhale. As you exhale, lean forward until you touch your forehead to the ground. Inhale and return to a sitting position. Repeat this process for several minutes.

For the next step, you will sit with your legs stretched out in front of you. Stretch forward and grab your toes. As you exhale, lengthen your spine. Remain in this position and breathe normally for several minutes.

In order to end this kriya, you will again sit in Easy Pose. Keep your spine straight and your palms resting on your knees.

Bring your right ear to your right shoulder. Slowly roll your head to the other side. Roll your neck in a gentle circular motion for one minute and then reverse directions. Roll your neck in the opposite direction for one minute and then relax.

Detoxification

The modern world is full of toxifying agents. From the food in the grocery stores to the air that we breathe. These toxins can have a profound impact on your overall health. This next kriya can help to detoxify your body.

Lie down on your back. Stretch your legs out with your heels together. Point your toes upward. While your heels are together, spread your feet apart so that they are pointing out to the sides. Then, close your feet so that the toes are pointing upwards again. Continue opening and closing your feet in this manner for several minutes.

Remain on your back. Place your hands under your head. Raise your legs about two feet off the ground. Move your legs in a scissor motion, but do not allow your heel to touch the ground. Keep your legs straight and do not bend your knees. Continue moving your legs in a scissor motion for 4 minutes.

Next, lie down on your stomach. Hold your head up and stick your tongue out. Take a deep breath. As you exhale, push yourself up to cobra position. For this pose, stretch your arms to lift your shoulders and upper body upward. Stretch your head and spine upward, like a cobra rising from the ground.

Inhale as you lower yourself back to the ground. Repeat this movement for 6 minutes. Exhale and rise to cobra pose and then inhale as you lower yourself back to the ground.

Next, turn over and lie on your back. Bring your knees up to your chest. Stretch your arms up towards the ceiling. Hold this pose for several seconds.

Stretch your legs back out in front of you and lower your arms at the same time. Repeat this movement of bringing your knees towards your chest and raising your arms for 3 minutes.

Sit in Easy Pose. Rotate your torso to the left and then to the right. Repeat this movement for 3 minutes.

Now, you can stand up. Bend over and touch your ankles. Hold on to your ankles and slowly sit down and then stand back up. Continue holding onto your ankles throughout this movement. Repeat this motion for 2 minutes.

Return to Easy Pose. Keep your spine straight. Take a deep breath and stretch your arms over your head. Touch your palms together. Hold your breath for about 40 seconds and then exhale. Repeat this twice more and then relax.

Energy

This next kriya is a short, simple kriya that can be performed to give yourself a boost of energy. You can perform this kriya several times per day to relieve stress, improve mental clarity, and give yourself some additional energy.

Sit on the floor with your legs stretched out in front of you. Lean forward and touch your toes. Stretch your nose towards your toes.

Hold this pose as you continue to breathe gently. Use a mantra to meditate on this pose for several minutes – or, up to 11 minutes.

That is all that is required for this kriya. You can perform this kriya several times per day. For example, you could do this in the morning, during your lunch break, and then when you get home from work.

Headaches

Headaches are a common problem and there are many home remedies. But, by performing this simple kriya, you can naturally cleanse your mind and free yourself of headaches.

This kriya can help stimulate your brain. This activity should be able to help alleviate your headache.

Lie on your back with your arms stretched on the floor above your head. Spread your legs wide apart on the floor. Once you are comfortable, inhale and sit up. Stretch your arms forward and touch your hands to the floor between your legs.

Exhale and lie back down. Repeat this 26 times. Be careful when sitting up, especially if you have a history of back problems.

Vitality

Increasing your vitality and stamina is the goal of this next kriya. This may be one of the most effective kriya for opening up the flow of energy and preventing blockages. Stand up with your feet about shoulder-width apart.

Bend down and touch your fingertips to the ground in front of you. Move your weight towards your hips as you balance on your toes and fingertips. This is similar to a downward facing dog, but with your fingertips closer to your legs.

Once you are comfortable with this position, begin moving your hips from side to side, like an animal wiggling its tail back and forth. Repeat this movement for 3 minutes.

Next, sit in Easy Pose. Lean backward, with your arms folded across your chest. Lock your elbows with your hands.

Continue leaning back until you are at a 60-degree angle. Keep your neck straight. You can pull your chin inward. Begin rolling your shoulders in a forward circle. Repeat this rolling motion for 3 minutes.

Lie down in the Baby Pose. For the Baby Pose, you will sit on your knees. Stretch forward, reaching your hands forward across the floor, until your forehead reaches the ground.

With your head still resting on the floor, lock your hands behind the small of your back. Interlock your finger and raise your arms behind your back and stretch them towards the ceiling. Hold this pose for 3 minutes.

Cross your legs into Lotus Pose. This basic pose is often used for meditation and as a starting point for other poses. First, sit on the floor with your legs extended in front of you. Your spine should be straight and your arms resting at your sides.

Bend your right knee and bring your right foot towards the crease of your left hip. Your right foot should rest on your left thigh, with you're the sole of your foot facing upwards. Repeat this process with your left leg, resting your left foot over your right thigh. This is the Lotus Pose.

Some people find it more comfortable to start with a specific leg. For example, you may find it easier to cross your right leg over your left thigh before crossing your left leg over your right thigh.

Next, you will place your arms behind you and lean backward until you are resting on your elbows. You will also hold this pose for 3 minutes.

Stretch your legs out in front of you. Next, grab your toes and bring your head towards your knees. Then, straighten back up. Repeat this movement 11 times. Breathe normally as you perform this motion.

For the final pose, sit in Easy Pose with your hands in prayer pose. Place your hands at the center of your chest. Close your eyes, keep your chin in and keep your neck straight. Pump your navel point for 3 minutes.

Inhale deeply and hold your breath as you tighten all of your muscles. Hold this for 10 seconds, exhale and repeat twice more. Afterward, relax your muscles and you are done with the kriya.

You can start using the kriyas described in this guide to improve your overall well-being and health. While each of these kriya has a specific purpose, they can all help to open the flow of energy and awaken Kundalini.

Review the various kriya presented in this guide and choose one or two that address issues you are currently dealing with. This could include the kriyas for headaches, anxiety, detoxification, or any of the other kriya provided. After you master the basics of these kriya, you can begin incorporating the other kriya from this guide.

Conclusion

Kundalini yoga should not be thought of as just an exercise or workout. It should become a part of your daily life. The kriya described in the previous chapter will only require 15 to 20 minutes out of your day. You should try to set aside some time each day to practice these kriyas, while also focusing on your breathing techniques and meditation.

The energy that you unleash will benefit you in every task. The calmness and sense of awareness you experience will help you succeed and reach your goals. These are benefits that you should continue to reap.

Continue practicing kundalini yoga on a regular basis. Make it a part of your life to improve your overall happiness and well-being. These are steps that anyone can take to improve their health and spiritual development.

Kundalini yoga is all about unleashing the energy that you already have while becoming more connected to the universal energy all around us. Hopefully, you will apply these tips and techniques to your daily life. You should start small, with one or two of the kriya mentioned in the previous chapter.

Also, remember to focus on your breathing techniques. Practice the breath of fire technique until you have mastered it. These breathing techniques and poses will help open up areas of your body that may not regularly receive enough attention.

You can breathe more life into your lungs, promote better blood circulation, and lower your heart rate. This all adds up to improved health and mental clarity.

"When your mind thinks too much, it loses touch with the reality of life. To be real, our feet should be on the Earth and our head should be in the Heavens." – Yogi Bhajan

Resources

Thank you for reading "Kundalini Yoga Meditation Awakening Guide for Beginners"! Did you enjoy reading this book? If so, please share a couple of sentences and a 4-5 star review on Amazon. It would mean a great deal to me and others who are looking.

If you have any questions or comments, feel free to email me at info@ sparrowpublications.com. I do my best reply to all questions that come in and that I am able to.

Sign up for updates of our new books, free bonuses and more...
www.sparrowpublications.com

Visit our store for yoga, natural health related products!
www.enaturestore.com

Subscribe to the Nature's Natural Health Newsletter and receive instant access to your FREE 28-page report: *"The Natural Strengthening Properties of Organic Healing: Heal Yourself With All Natural Organic Power"* Continue here to get your report now!

www.naturesnaturalhealth.com/join/

www.ingramcontent.com/pod-product-compliance
Lightning Source LLC
Chambersburg PA
CBHW070247290526
45789CB00004B/1799